NUTRITION FOR WEIGHT LOSS SURGERY

# Shopping Companion

## JUSTINE HAWKE & SALLY JOHNSTON

ACCREDITED PRACTISING DIETITIANS | ACCREDITED NUTRITIONISTS

# Contents

Navigating the supermarket and the ever-growing range of products available can be an enormous challenge. Many of our patients feel overwhelmed as they try to make the best choices and end up feeling lost and confused. That is why we have done the hard work for you and developed the 'Weight Loss Surgery Shopping Companion'.

This shopping companion steps you through a wide range of product categories to help you decide on the best choices for your requirements post weight loss surgery.

The products most suited to post weight loss surgery requirements are typically rich in good quality protein, high in fibre, not too high in fat, sugar or salt. They are therefore great choices for everyone, not just those that have had weight loss surgery.

It is important to remember that the examples given throughout the guide are just some of the options available. There may be products that are not listed that are also suitable.

**Don't forget to check your favourite brands and varieties against our selection criteria to see how closely they fit.**

**Our 'selection criteria' is just a guideline and doesn't have to be used as a strict rule.**

It is important to note, not all supermarkets stock all product lines and some products in our top pick list are available online only. If you can't find one of our top picks at your local store, it can be useful to look online to find your nearest stockist.

It is also important to remember that products change, packaging may be updated and some of our 'top picks' may become discontinued. We endeavor to keep this shopping companion as up to date as possible and welcome feedback anytime via our social media platforms.

The information in this guide was correct at the time of printing and there has been no financial incentive to list any of the products highlighted in our top picks list.

**Throughout the guide we compare foods per 100g, or occasionally, per serve. We must stress however, that when using this guide, always remember to judge the portion you choose to eat based on your individual capacity, always stopping when you are satisfied, not full.**

Before jumping into the selection criteria, we wanted to start by giving you some simple tips and tricks that may help you with your weekly shop. Many people skip these steps and end up with a trolley packed with food items they didn't plan to purchase and may not necessarily be what they need to put their meals together for the week.

The most important thing you can do before you shop is to plan your meals for the week. Our Nutrition for Weight Loss Surgery Meal Plans are a great place to start and are available via our online store at: www.nfwls.com

When planning your meals, remember to include your three core meals as well as snacks (if needed). It is fine to repeat meals, for example, you may be happy to have the same breakfast seven mornings per week, or enjoy the same morning snack every workday. Think about what is happening in your week. What nights will you arrive home late? What meal preparation time will you have? What day will you need to pop the slow cooker on, or have a quick, easy option ready to go?

As you only need smaller meals post surgery, try to make the most of your cooking time and cook extra portions to freeze or use as leftovers for lunch.

Based on your meal plan, write your shopping list. But more importantly, take that list with you! Try to stick to the list as closely as you can. This will help with your budget as well as your health goals.

Before heading to the supermarket be sure to have a meal or snack. Hunger makes us much more vulnerable to impulse purchases, so safe guard yourself against this.

If you find you are always tempted by the 'special buys' on display, are succumbing to 'pester power' or just don't have the time you need to make good choices at the supermarket, perhaps you should try online shopping. It certainly makes sticking to the list a little easier.

## FRESH IS BEST

This guide is designed to help you navigate the packaged products available throughout the supermarket, however, try to make fresh foods the focus of your shopping. Fill your trolley with lean proteins, fruits, vegetables, grains, legumes and dairy products. They have minimal processing and don't have long ingredient lists for you to interpret. Choose whole, fresh, real food wherever possible.

This isn't to say there isn't a place for some packaged food, but the bulk of what you eat post surgery should be focused on uncomplicated, minimally processed proteins, balanced with vegetables or salads, some grains, dairy and healthy fats. Formulated protein bars, balls, shakes or puddings shouldn't replace real food long term.

In an ideal world we would love to see you doing regular weekly meal planning. However, we know that the best laid plans don't always fall into place.

To safe guard yourself from falling into grabbing snacks from the service station on the way to work, or swinging into the drive through on the way home, you want to be equipped with a well-stocked fridge and pantry. It should be filled with items that allow you to quickly pull together a nutritious breakfast, quick snack or no fuss meal.

Our suggested pantry staples include the following.

### FRIDGE:

- milk or protein rich milk alternatives such as soy milk
- Greek yoghurt (as this is the most versatile, appropriate for sweet and savoury purposes)
- hard cheese
- ricotta or cottage cheese
- eggs
- chutney or relish
- fresh fruit and vegetables
- pickled vegetables such as chargrilled capsicum, gherkins, olives, sauerkraut and red cabbage.

### FREEZER:

- frozen vegetables
- frozen fruit
- individual meat, poultry or fish portions
- individual portions of leftovers labeled and dated.

### PANTRY:

- oats
- canned fish such as salmon and tuna
- canned legumes and lentils including four bean mix, chickpeas and lentils
- canned vegetables including tomatoes and corn
- nuts and seeds
- grainy crackers
- rice, including instant brown or black rice
- instant quinoa
- pasta
- dried herbs and spices
- olive oil
- vinegar(s)
- nut paste, such as peanut or almond paste
- dried fruit such as dates or dried apricots
- salsa.

Our selection criteria refers to the nutrition information panel. However, it is also important to check the ingredient list, as this gives you a clear picture of what is in the food you are choosing to eat.

If you want to avoid artificial sweeteners, additives, preservatives or have an allergy or intolerance, it is essential you review the ingredient list to see if it is a product suitable for you to include.

Ingredients are listed in order from the highest to lowest content in the food. If fat or sugar (or one of the clever names also meaning fat, salt or sugar, see list below) are in the first few ingredients on the list, take care.

| FAT | SUGAR | SALT |
|---|---|---|
| animal fat | fructose | salt |
| shortening | lactose | sodium |
| beef fat | honey | rock salt |
| lard | sucrose | sea salt |
| dripping | sugar, raw sugar | onion salt |
| cream | invert sugar | celery salt |
| butter, butter fat | glucose syrup | garlic salt |
| tallow | malt, malt extract | booster |
| coconut oil | dextrose | MSG (monosodium glutamate) |
| palm oil | treacle | meat/vegetable extract |
| vegetable fat | golden syrup | stock cubes |
| chocolate | molasses | sodium bicarbonate |
| monoglycerides | maple syrup | baking powder |
| milk solids | glucose syrup | sodium metabisulphite |
| hydrogenated oils | brown sugar | vegetable salt |
| margarine | corn syrup | yeast extracts |
| chocolate or carob coating | concentrated fruit juice | kosher salt |
| seeds, nuts & coconut | maltose | pink Himalayan salt |
| oil | modified carbohydrate | sodium nitrate |
| copha | agave nectar/syrup | sodium citrate |
| diglycerides | barley malt | sodium chloride |
| cocoa butter | beet sugar | sodium diacetate |
| | carob syrup | sodium erythorbate |
| | coconut sugar | sodium glutamate |
| | coffee sugar crystals | sodium lactate |
| | fruit juice | sodium lauryl sulfate |
| | high fructose corn syrup (HFCS) | sodium phosphate |
| | palm sugar | trisodium phosphate |
| | rice syrup | |
| | icing sugar | |
| | corn sweetener | |

# Selection Criteria:
# Grains

........................

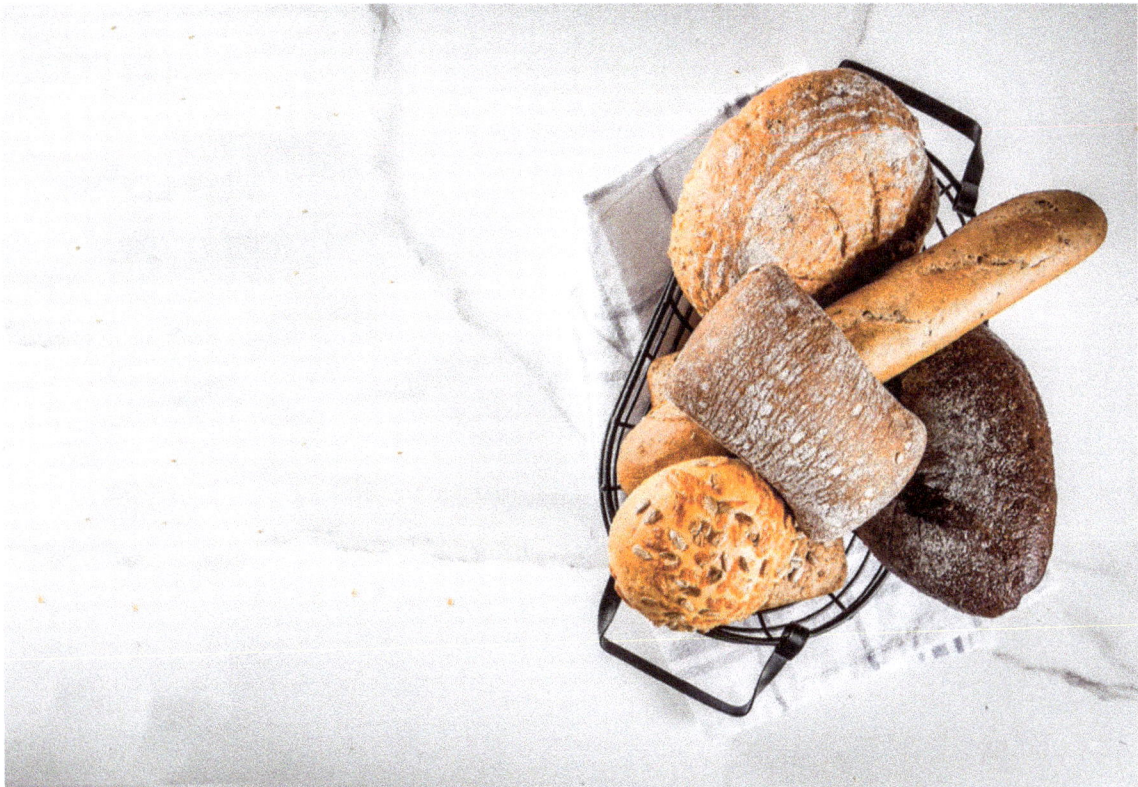

# Bread

A good quality, high fibre bread can be included in your diet following weight loss surgery.

You may find toasted bread easier to tolerate than fresh, and often one slice (or less) is enough.

Surprisingly some breads have more protein per slice than an egg, so can help you to reach your protein needs. Wholegrain breads are also an excellent way to boost your fibre intake.

As bread is portion controlled, we suggest you look per slice.

### WHEN CHOOSING BREAD, LOOK FOR OPTIONS THAT HAVE:

- Less than 20g of total carbohydrate per slice
- Greater than 3g protein per slice
- Less than 5g total fat per slice
- Greater than 3g fibre per slice
- Less than 400mg sodium per 100g.

### OUR TOP PICKS INCLUDE:

- Aldi 85% Less Carb, High Protein Bread *
- Bakers Delight, Cape Seed Loaf**
- Helgas Lower Carb, Wholemeal and Seed
- Helga's Wholemeal Grain
- Herman Brot Lower Carb Bread*
- Tip Top 9 Grain Wholemeal.

* High protein low, carbohydrate breads are higher in fat than our selection criteria. However, due to the low carbohydrate content they are an excellent product to include, particularly if you require a low carbohydrate diet.

** Slightly higher than our selection criteria for fat.

# Wraps and Flat Bread

A well selected wrap or flat bread is a versatile addition to your shopping list.

It can make a simple base for your lunch when filled with lean protein and salad, toasted with your favourite filling or topped to make a quick 'cheats pizza'. You can even toast wraps in your oven and serve as an alternative to crackers or corn chips with high protein dips.

Care must be taken when choosing wraps or flat bread as some options contain as much carbohydrate as three or more slices of bread. It is therefore worth becoming familiar with the following selection criteria before your next shop.

### NFWLS SELECTION CRITERIA

As wraps and flatbreads are portion controlled, we suggest you look per serve.

### WHEN CHOOSING A WRAP OR FLAT BREAD, LOOK FOR OPTIONS THAT HAVE:

- Less than 20g of total carbohydrate per wrap
- Greater than 3g protein per wrap
- Less than 5g total fat per wrap
- Greater than 3g fibre per wrap
- Less than 400mg sodium per 100g

### OUR TOP PICKS INCLUDE:

- Abbotts Village Bakery, Sandwich Thins, Mixed Seeds and Grains
- BFree Quinoa & Chia Seed Wraps*
- Freedom Foods Barley + Whole Grain Barley Wraps
- Helga's Lower Carb Wholemeal Wraps*
- Mission Low Carb Wraps*
- Tip Top Sandwich Thins, Wholemeal.

* Slightly higher than our selection criteria for sodium.

# Crackers and Crispbread

Some people find crackers and crispbreads easier to tolerate than bread following weight loss surgery.

Like most foods, there are some fabulous choices, but also some options that are not particularly nutritious.

No matter which cracker or crispbread option you select, be mindful of your portions, as they can be very easy to over eat.

NFWLS SELECTION CRITERIA

WHEN CHOOSING CRACKERS OR CRISPBREAD, LOOK FOR OPTIONS THAT HAVE:

- Greater than 6g protein per 100g
- Greater than 6g fibre per 100g
- Less than 10g fat per 100g
- Less than 400mg sodium per 100g.

OUR TOP PICKS INCLUDE:

- Arnott's Vita-Weat*
- Carman's Super Seed and Grain Crackers, Ancient Grain and Cracked Pepper**
- Real Foods Multigrain and Soy & Linseed Corn Thins
- Ryvita Multigrain and Original.

* Slightly higher than our selection criteria for sodium.

** Carman's Super Seed and Grain Crackers are higher in fat than our selection criteria. However, due to the very low carbohydrate content, they are still an excellent product to include, particularly if you require a low carbohydrate diet.

# Breakfast Cereal

Breakfast cereal can be an excellent inclusion in your post surgery diet, however it can also be a hidden source of excess sugars and fats if not selected carefully.

It can also be very easy to overdo your portion, as when served with milk it is easily tolerated post weight loss surgery.

To help control your portion, serve your cereal using a half cup measure, which provides a similar amount of carbohydrate to one slice of bread. If this doesn't feel enough, use some good quality yoghurt (see page 26) and/or fruit to make it more satisfying.

## NFWLS SELECTION CRITERIA

### WHEN CHOOSING A BREAKFAST CEREAL, LOOK FOR OPTIONS THAT HAVE:

- Greater than 8g protein per 100g
- Greater than 8g fibre per 100g
- Less than 15g sugar per 100g
- Less than 10g total fat per 100g
- Less than 400mg sodium per 100g.

### OUR TOP PICKS INCLUDE:

- Be Natural, 5 Whole Grain Flakes
- Freedom Foods, Active Balance Buckwheat and Quinoa
- Kellogg's Guardian Cereal
- Special K Nourish, Blackcurrant, Apple and Pepita*
- Uncle Tobys Bran Plus.

* Slightly higher than our selection criteria for sugar.

# Muesli and Granola

The selection criteria for muesli and granola are different to the criteria for breakfast cereals. As muesli and granola contain more nuts and seeds, the fat content of these is generally slightly higher. This can help you feel satisfied for longer.

Like breakfast cereals, it is important to control your portion, so using a quarter cup measure can be useful. This will provide a similar amount of carbohydrate to one slice of bread.

WHEN CHOOSING A MUESLI OR GRANOLA, LOOK FOR OPTIONS THAT HAVE:

- Greater than 8g protein per 100g
- Greater than 8g fibre per 100g
- Less than 15g sugar per 100g
- Less than 25g total fat per 100g
- Less than 3g saturated fat per 100g
- Less than 400mg sodium per 100g.

OUR TOP PICKS INCLUDE:

- Freedom Foods Barley + Barley Clusters*
- Freedom Foods Barley + Protein Clusters*
- Carman Original Fruit Free Muesli
- Carman's Honey Roasted Nut Crunchy Clusters
- Food for Health Chia & Cinnamon Fruit Free Clusters
- Food for Health Liver Cleansing Muesli
- Jordans Low Sugar Granola, Almond and Hazelnut
- Lowan Original Harvest Muesli
- Table of Plenty, Nicely Nutty Fruit Free Muesli
- Woolworths Great Start Protein Clusters.

*Slightly higher than our selection criteria for sugar.

# Porridge and Oats

Nutritionally, the best type of porridge is good old-fashioned oats. However, the flavoured options are tasty, quick and easy, hence very popular.

Care needs to be taken as some of these options are loaded with sugar, so use our selection criteria to help guide your choice.

NFWLS SELECTION CRITERIA

WHEN CHOOSING PORRIDGE OR OATS, LOOK FOR OPTIONS THAT HAVE:

- Greater than 8g protein per 100g
- Greater than 8g fibre per 100g
- Less than 15g sugar per 100g
- Less than 10g total fat per 100g
- Less than 400mg sodium per 100g.

OUR TOP PICKS INCLUDE:

- Carman's Gourmet Porridge Sachets, Honey, Vanilla and Cinnamon
- Carman's Gourmet Porridge Sachets, Super Berry & Coconut
- Heritage Mill Porridge Sachets, range
- Macro Organic Quick Oats
- Orgran Brekki Quinoa Porridge, Berry
- Uncle Tobys Quick Oat Sachets, Original
- Uncle Tobys Quick Oat Sachets, High Fibre
- Uncle Tobys Oats Super Blends Protein.

# Breakfast Cereal Biscuits

Breakfast cereal biscuits are a staple in many homes.

One of the advantages of them is they are portion controlled. Following weight loss surgery most people can tolerate between half and up to two biscuits.

There are new products in this range hitting the market and the following selection criteria can help you to determine if they are a good choice for you.

WHEN CHOOSING A BREAKFAST CEREAL BISCUIT, LOOK FOR OPTIONS THAT HAVE:

- Greater than 8g protein per 100g
- Greater than 8g fibre per 100g
- Less than 15g sugar per 100g
- Less than 10g total fat per 100g
- Less than 400mg sodium per 100g,

OUR TOP PICKS INCLUDE:

- Coles Wheat Biscuits, Low Sugar
- Sanitarium Weet-Bix Gluten Free*
- Sanitarium Weet-Bix Original
- Sanitarium Weet-Bix Blends, Multi-Grain +
- Uncle Tobys Oat Brits
- Uncle Tobys VitaBrits No Added Sugar
- Woolworths Wheat Biscuits.

*Slightly lower than our selection criteria for fibre.

# Rice and Rice Blends (including instant varieties)

Rice and rice blends are a suitable accompaniment to many dishes and do not have to be avoided post weight loss surgery.

As with other carbohydrate foods, the key is controlling the portion you consume. One third of a cup of cooked rice provides approximately the same amount of carbohydrate as an average slice of bread.

Keep in mind that rice can swell in your stomach, so take care to eat slowly and stop at satisfied, not full.

If you choose to avoid rice, alternatives such as cauliflower or broccoli 'rice' are an excellent substitute.

Look for low glycemic index (low GI) rice. Low GI foods are digested slower and help to keep you feeling fuller for longer.

## OPTIONS INCLUDE:

- Basmati
- Sunrice Doongara Clever Rice
- Wild rice.

If you prefer other rice varieties, try to select those with as much fibre and protein as possible.

## NFWLS SELECTION CRITERIA

### WHEN CHOOSING RICE OR RICE BLEND, LOOK FOR OPTIONS THAT HAVE:

- Greater than 4g protein per 100g
- Greater than 3g fibre per 100g.

## OUR TOP PICKS INCLUDE:

- Coles 7 Ancient Grains Microwave Rice
- Riviana Brown Basmati Rice
- Sunrice Black Rice
- Sunrice SuperGrains, Active Blend Microwave Rice*.

## STANDOUT PRODUCT

A standout product in this category is The Protein Bread Co P300 Protein Rice. It is a blend of lupin, brown and black rice, providing 31g of protein and 20g fibre per 100g. This is available online via:

www.theproteinbreadco.com.au

*Slightly below our selection criteria for fibre.

# Pasta and Noodles

Pasta and noodles can still be enjoyed post weight loss surgery, as long as they do not replace the protein and vegetable portion of your meals on a regular basis.

As with other carbohydrate foods, the key is controlling the portion you consume. Half a cup of cooked standard wheat pasta provides approximately the same amount of carbohydrate as an average slice of bread.

If you prefer to avoid noodles and pasta, you could consider using low calorie alternatives like konjac noodles (for example Slendier Slim Noodles) or zucchini noodles.

If you are looking for pasta with added nutritional benefits, there are some products with extra protein and fibre to look out for.

The following selection criteria will make it easier for you to spot these higher protein and fibre options.

## NFWLS SELECTION CRITERIA

### WHEN CHOOSING PASTA OR NOODLES, LOOK FOR OPTIONS THAT HAVE:

- Greater than 6g protein per 100g
- Greater than 4g fibre per 100g
- Less than 5g total fat per 100g
- Less than 400mg sodium per 100g.

### OUR TOP PICKS INCLUDE:

- Herman Brot Lower Carb Pasta
- San Remo Pulse Pasta
- San Remo Wholemeal Lasagna Sheets
- San Remo Wholemeal Spirals
- Vetta Smart Pasta, High Protein, Low Carb.

Other grain foods that meet our selection criteria for both rice and pasta include barley, buckwheat, bulgur (cracked wheat), freekeh, millet and quinoa. Be sure to consider these grains as alternatives to rice and pasta in your dishes.

*Slightly higher than our selection criteria for fat.

# Selection Criteria:
# Meat & Meat Alternatives

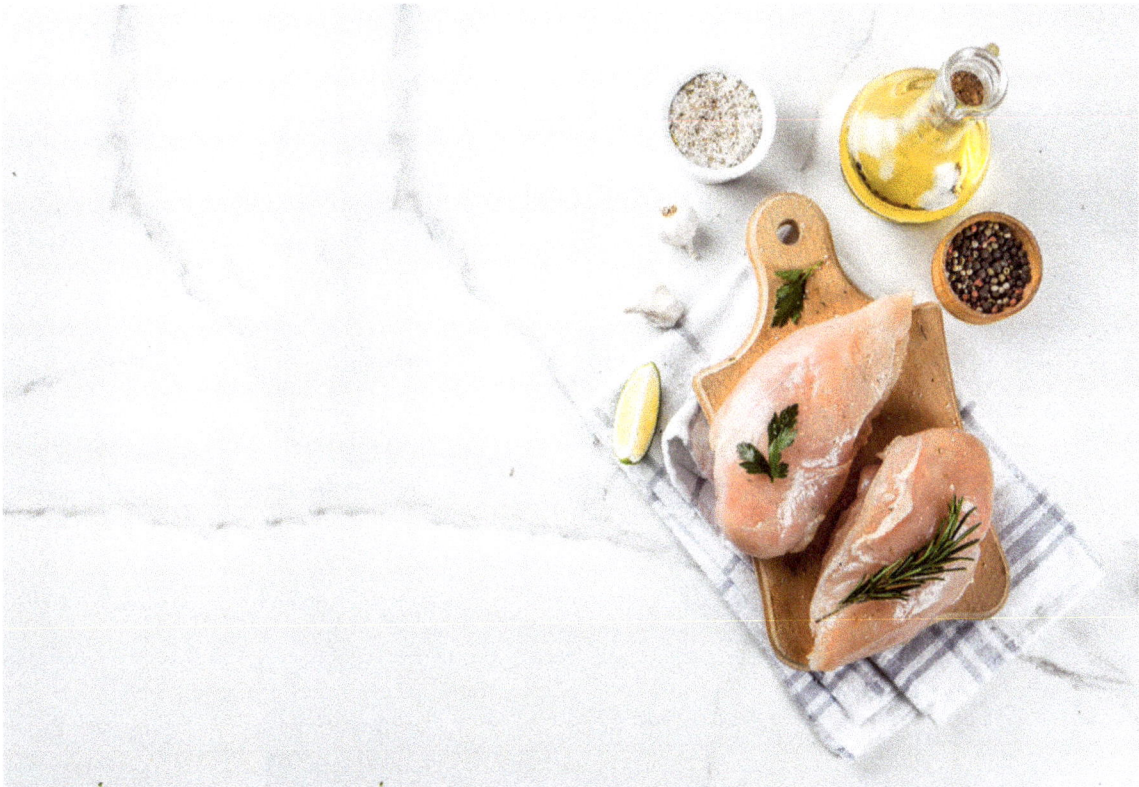

# Deli and Pre Cooked Meats

Whilst pre cooked meats are convenient and popular, many options are high in sodium and saturated fat and not always a good source of high quality protein.

When it comes to protein, fresh is best.

When using your oven or barbeque, grill some chicken tenderloins to add to wraps, sandwiches and salads, or use leftover roast meats in place of processed deli sliced options.

If you do choose precooked deli meats, the following selection criteria can help guide you on better options.

WHEN CHOOSING DELI AND PRE COOKED MEATS, LOOK FOR OPTIONS THAT HAVE:

- Greater than 10g protein per 100g
- Less than 10g carbohydrate per 100g
- Less than 10g total fat per 100g
- Less than 3g saturated fat per 100g
- Less than 400mg sodium per 100g.

OUR TOP PICKS INCLUDE:

- Coles Sliced Roast Chicken Breast, Peri Peri
- Three Aussie Farmers Slow Cooked & Pulled Roast Chicken with Chicken Seasoning
- Moira Mac's Homestyle Chicken Breast Slices
- Moira Mac's Sliced Chicken Breast, Tandoori.

# Frozen Chicken, Fish and Seafood Products

Whilst fresh is best, the wide range of processed frozen chicken, fish and seafood products available in the supermarket clearly shows how popular these are.

We always recommend choosing unprocessed, fresh produce as often as possible. However, if you do choose to have some processed frozen chicken, fish or seafood it is best to use the following criteria to help select the more nutritious varieties.

NFWLS SELECTION CRITERIA

WHEN CHOOSING FROZEN CHICKEN, FISH AND SEAFOOD PRODUCTS, LOOK FOR OPTIONS THAT HAVE:

- Greater than 20g protein per 100g
- Less than 10g carbohydrate per 100g
- Less than 10g total fat per 100g
- Less than 3g saturated fat per 100g
- Less than 400mg sodium per 100g.

OUR TOP CHICKEN PICKS INCLUDE:

- Created with Jamie Crumbed Chicken Range
- Ingham's Free Range Chicken Tenderloins Wholemeal and Quinoa*
- Lilydale Free Range Chicken Schnitzels, Herb Ciabatta**.

OUR TOP FISH AND SEAFOOD PICKS INCLUDE:

- Birds Eye Ocean Selections NZ Wild Caught Fillets, Hoki
- Birds Eye Ocean Selections NZ Wild Caught Fillets, Whiting*
- By George Australian Whole Cooked Tiger Prawns
- Just Caught Altantic Salmon, Skinless*
- Ocean Chef Salmon Portions, Skin On***
- Ocean Chef Yellowfin Tuna Steaks
- Pacific West Yellowfin Tuna Steaks.

*Slightly below our selection criteria for protein.
** Slightly below our selection criteria for protein and above our selection criteria for sodium.
*** Slightly above our selection criteria for fat.

# Tinned Fish

Tinned fish, including tuna, salmon and sardines are excellent pantry staples and add good quality protein to your diet.

Traditionally we have suggested tinned fish in spring water. However, a little good quality fat, such as tuna in olive oil, can help you feel more satisfied and improve your absorption of fat soluble vitamins. So don't feel these have to be avoided, simply drain off the excess oil.

NFWLS SELECTION CRITERIA

WHEN CHOOSING TINNED FISH PRODUCTS, LOOK FOR OPTIONS THAT HAVE:

- Greater than 20g protein per 100g
- Less than 10g carbohydrate per 100g
- Less than 10g total fat per 100g
- Less than 3g saturated fat per 100g
- Less than 400mg sodium per 100g.

OUR TOP PICKS INCLUDE:

- Coles Pink Salmon
- Greenseas Tuna Chunks in Spring Water
- John West Pink Salmon
- John West Salmon Slices in Spring Water
- John West Sardines in Spring Water*
- John West Tuna in Spring Water
- Safcol Responsibly Fished Tuna in oil
- Sirena Tuna in Spring Water
- Sirena Tuna in Oil with Lemon Pepper**
- Woolworths Select Pink Salmon
- Woolworths Yellowfin Tuna in Spring Water.

* Slightly below our selection criteria for protein, and above our criteria for fat.
** Slightly above our selection criteria for sodium.

# Sausages, Burgers and Patties

Sausages, burgers and patties are a barbeque favourite, but are typically high in fat, saturated fat and salt.

There is however some lean, lower sodium options available that are superior nutritionally.

It is important to ensure your choice also provides a significant source of protein.

The following selection criteria can help guide you.

NFWLS SELECTION CRITERIA

WHEN CHOOSING SAUSAGES, BURGERS AND PATTIES, LOOK FOR OPTIONS THAT HAVE:

- Greater than 10g protein per 100g
- Less than 10g carbohydrate per 100g
- Less than 10g total fat per 100g
- Less than 3g saturated fat per 100g
- Less than 400mg sodium per 100g.

OUR TOP PICKS INCLUDE:

- Grasslands Grass Fed Beef Burgers
- Ingham's Extra Lean Turkey Burgers*
- K Roo Kangaroo Sausages, Bush Tomato*
- Peppercorn Beef Burger, Extra Lean**
- Peppercorn Extra Lean Beef Sausages**.

* Higher in sodium than our selection criteria, not suitable on a low salt diet.
** Slightly higher in sodium than our selection criteria.

# Vegetarian Proteins (including Tofu and Tempeh)

For both vegetarians and non-vegetarians wanting to include more meat free options, it is important to look for protein rich alternatives to animal protein foods.

Some meat alternatives are low in protein, making it difficult to meet your minimum daily targets.

The following selection criteria can help guide you.

WHEN CHOOSING VEGETARIAN PROTEIN, LOOK FOR OPTIONS THAT HAVE:

- Greater than 15g protein per 100g
- Less than 10g carbohydrate per 100g
- Less than 10g total fat per 100g
- Less than 3g saturated fat per 100g
- Less than 400mg sodium per 100g.

OUR TOP PICKS INCLUDE:

- Coles Hard Tofu
- Linda McCartney's Vegetarian Sausages *
- Macro Textured Vegetable Protein
- Nutrisoy Organic Tasty Tempeh
- Nutrisoy Spicy Tofu
- Quorn Frozen Meat Free, Soy Free Mince
- Simply Better Plain Firm Tofu
- Soyco Spicy Thai Tofu
- Vegie Delights, Nutmeat*.

Whilst they do not meet the selection criteria above, chickpeas, lentils, kidney beans, butter beans, cannellini beans and other legumes are all excellent choices nutritionally, along with salt reduced baked beans. They provide an excellent source of low GI carbohydrate, fibre and protein, and can confidently be included in your diet.

* Above our selection criteria for sodium, not suitable on a low salt diet
** Slightly above our selection criteria for fat

# Selection Criteria:
# Dairy & Alternatives

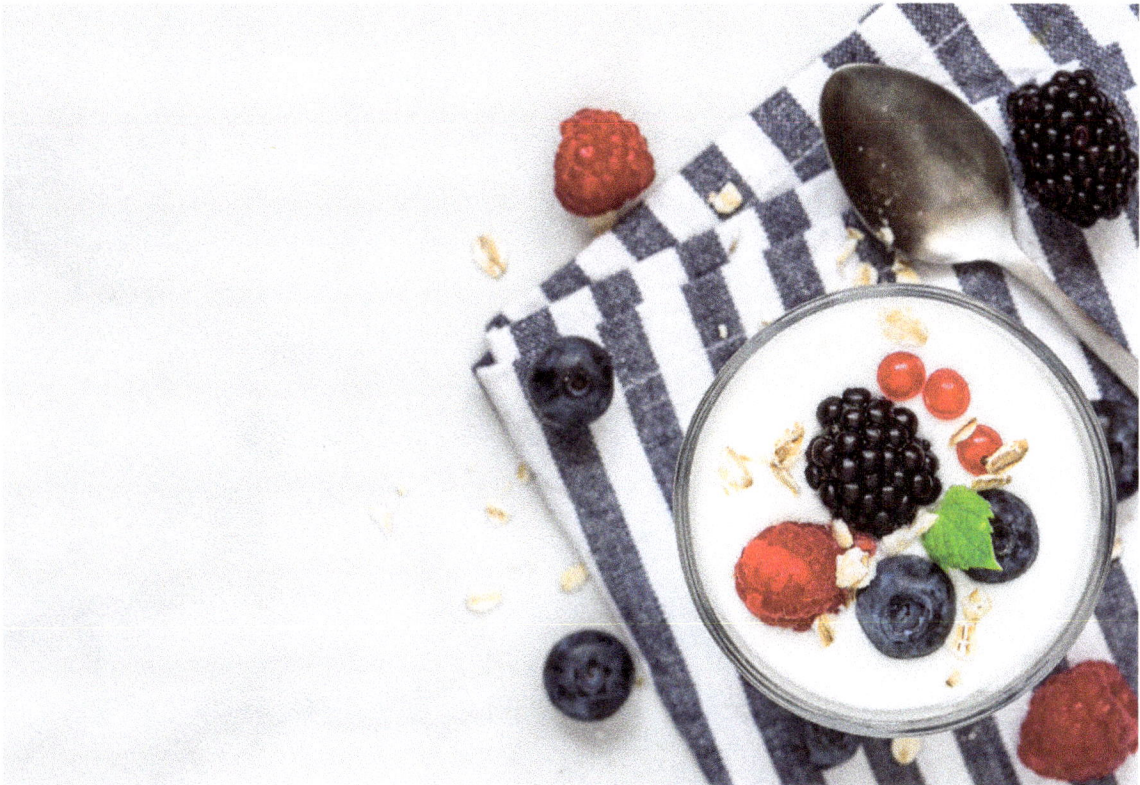

# Milk

Cow's milk is a wonderful source of nutrition rich in protein, vitamins and minerals.

Unless you are drinking large amounts every day, our advice is select what you enjoy.

If you are using a lot of milk and trying to keep your overall energy intake low, selecting a lower fat variety can help with this.

Some people tend to avoid lower fat varieties, believing they are higher in sugar. This is not because sugar has been added to the milk, but because the concentration of natural sugar (lactose) becomes higher when fat is removed.

The protein content of full cream, reduced fat, light and skim milks varies from about 3.3 – 3.9g per 100g. Therefore there is no reason to select a particular type of milk due to its protein content.

## STANDOUT PRODUCT

A standout product in this category is The Complete Dairy High Protein Milk. This provides almost double the amount of protein of standard milks, at 6g protein per 100g. This is therefore an excellent choice if you find it difficult to meet your protein targets.

# Cow's Milk Alternatives

A good quality milk alternative should be a significant source of both protein and calcium. The issue with many milk alternatives is that they are low in both of these.

Some options can also have excess added sugars, so it is important to look out for this too.

To help you choose the best option, the following selection criteria can be helpful.

## NFWLS SELECTION CRITERIA

### WHEN CHOOSING MILK ALTERNATIVES, LOOK FOR OPTIONS THAT HAVE:

- Greater than 3g protein per 100g
- Less than 5g sugar per 100g
- Added calcium.

### OUR TOP PICKS INCLUDE:

- Australia's Own, Like Milk
- Australia's Own, Unsweetened Like Milk
- Coles Regular Soy Milk
- Macro Organic Creamy Soy Milk
- Sanitarium So Good Soy Milk
- Vitasoy Calci Plus Soy Milk
- Vitasoy Unsweetened Soy Milk Protein Plus.

# Yoghurt

Yoghurt is a fabulous fridge staple and makes not only a perfect snack, but can be a great addition to breakfast, a protein boost to smoothies, a great base for dips and dressings and a sour cream alternative.

After weight loss surgery we encourage you to choose a higher protein option that tastes great. There is no need to stick to the ultra low fat or 'diet' varieties.

A well stocked fridge should contain both plain, Greek yoghurt, due to its versatility, as well as some 'grab and go' flavoured options for a nutrient rich snack.

NFWLS SELECTION CRITERIA

WHEN CHOOSING YOGHURT, LOOK FOR OPTIONS THAT HAVE:

- Greater than 5g protein per 100g
- Less than 10g sugar per 100g
- Less than 2g fat per 100g.

OUR TOP PICKS INCLUDE:

- Aldi Dairy Dream Hi-Protein Natural Yoghurt
- Chobani Plain, Flavoured and Fit yoghurt ranges*
- Danone YoPro range
- Farmers Union, Greek Style, Less than 0.5% fat yoghurt
- Woolworths Icelandic Style Skyr Yoghurt range.

*The Chobani Flip range is higher in sugar than our selection criteria.

# Cottage and Cream Cheese

Soft spreadable cheeses like cottage and cream cheese are great to spread on crackers, to use as a dip with vegetable sticks and in cooking to add creaminess or a cheesy flavor.

When selecting these types of soft cheese, try to choose options with as much protein and little fat as possible, and watch the sodium content.

NFWLS SELECTION CRITERIA

WHEN CHOOSING A SOFT SPREADABLE CHEESE, LOOK FOR OPTIONS THAT HAVE:

- Greater than 10g protein per 100g
- Less than 10g carbohydrate per 100g
- Less than 10g total fat per 100g
- Less than 3g saturated fat per 100g
- Less than 400mg sodium per 100g.

OUR TOP PICKS INCLUDE:

- Brancourts Classic Cottage Cheese
- Brancourts Protein + Cottage Cheese
- Bulla Low Fat, High Protein Cottage Cheese
- Philadelphia Protein Spreadable Cream Cheese*
- Woolworths Creamed Cottage Cheese.

Whilst reduced fat ricotta cheese is useful in cooking, it does not meet our criteria for protein. Be sure to account for this elsewhere in your day if including a ricotta based dish.

*Slightly higher saturated fat than our selection criteria.

# Other Cheeses

Cheese is a popular snack choice post weight loss surgery. It can also be a great way to sneak some extra protein into your meals by adding it to salads, grating over vegetables and adding into your cooking.

Although it is a great source of protein, cheese is typically a high saturated fat and high salt food. This doesn't mean it has to be avoided, but rather care must be taken with portions.

A portion or serve of cheese is approximately 40g, so try to limit your maximum daily intake to this.

The below table will help you compare the protein, fat and sodium content of a variety of cheeses to help you select the variety that best meets your needs.

## CHEESE COMPARISON CHART

| CHEESE | PROTEIN PER 40G SERVE | FAT PER 40G SERVE | SODIUM PER 40G SERVE |
| --- | --- | --- | --- |
| Blue Vein | 8g | 13g | 436mg |
| Bocconcini | 7g | 8g | 140mg |
| Brie | 8g | 13g | 244mg |
| Camembert | 8g | 10g | 244mg |
| Cheddar | 10g | 13g | 274mg |
| Feta | 7g | 8g | 480mg |
| Gouda | 10g | 12g | 280mg |
| Haloumi | 9g | 7g | 1160mg |

# Ice Cream And Dairy Desserts

The ever-expanding range of ice cream and dairy dessert options is appealing to those looking for a sweet indulgence.

Some products are low in sugar and fat and high in protein when compared to standard ice creams or dairy desserts, making them a better choice.

Just remember to watch the portion size as ice cream and dairy desserts are very easy to overeat, even after weight loss surgery.

The following selection criteria can help guide your choice.

NFWLS SELECTION CRITERIA

WHEN CHOOSING AN ICE CREAM OR DAIRY DESSERT, LOOK FOR OPTIONS THAT HAVE:

- Greater than 5g protein per 100g
- Less than 10g sugar per 100g
- Less than 8g fat per 100g.

OUR TOP PICKS INCLUDE:

- FroPro range
- Halo Top range*
- Tilly's Guilt Free Frozen Dessert *
- WheyWhip range.

* Slightly higher than our selection criteria for sugar in some flavours.

# Selection Criteria:
# Fats & Oils

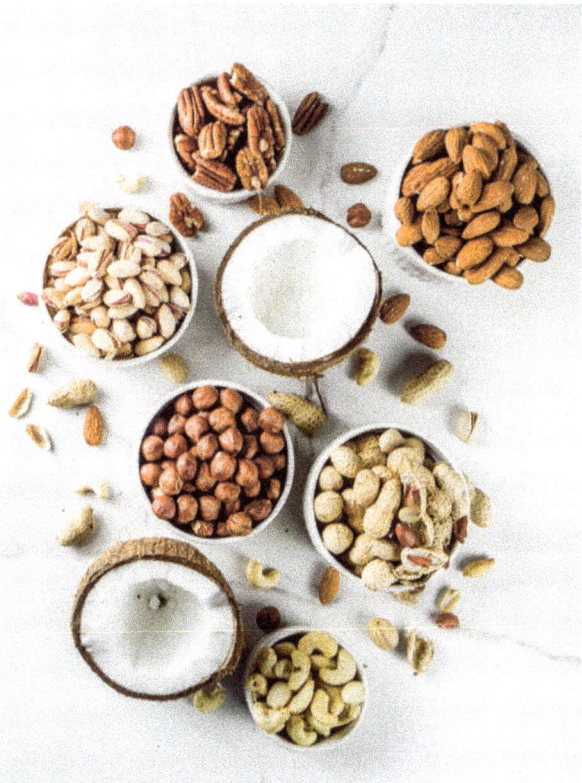

# Oils and Spreads

As most oils and spreads are purely fat, choosing on fat content alone is not appropriate.

It is however important to choose those lower in saturated fat, therefore making them higher in unsaturated fats, to promote good heart health.

Following is the saturated fat content of some oils and spreads, per 100g:

- Canola 7g
- Safflower 9g
- Sunflower 11g
- Olive 15g
- Peanut 18g
- Sesame 15g
- Soybean 15g
- Rice bran 23g
- Butter 53g
- Ghee 65g
- Coconut 85-95g.

Keep in mind that, even healthy fats need to be consumed in small amounts. For example, after weight loss surgery, many people may only need the equivalent of a couple of tablespoons of fat per day from all of their food. You can find more details on how much fat you require in our Weight Loss Surgery Meal Plans, available at:

www.nfwls.com.

# Nuts and Seeds

Nuts and seeds are a great source of protein and heart healthy fats.

The best option is plain, unflavoured varieties. If you enjoy salted nuts, combine one salted variety with three to four unsalted varieties to lower the sodium content.

When including nuts and seeds as a snack, limit your serve to 30 – 40g. However, this may be too much if you also use oils, spreads and avocado regularly, so consider your total fat intake over the day.

The protein content of nuts and seeds varies. The list below indicate the protein content of nuts per 40g serve:

| <5G PROTEIN PER 40G | 5-10G PROTEIN PER 40G | >10G PROTEIN PER 40G |
|---|---|---|
| macadamias | almonds | hemp seeds |
| pecans | brazil nuts | pumpkin seeds (pepitas) |
| | cashews | sunflower seeds |
| | chia seeds | |
| | flaxseeds | |
| | pine nuts | |
| | pistachios | |
| | walnuts | |

## NUT PASTES AND BUTTERS

Good quality nut pastes and butters can be spread on grainy crackers and bread, scraped onto celery or vegetable sticks, added to smoothies or used in salad dressings and marinades.

What makes a nut paste a good choice is what is not added to it. Try to select nut pastes and butters without added sugars, additives and preservatives. When looking at a nut paste or butter, check the ingredients list. The fewer ingredients you find, the better.

## OUR TOP PICKS INCLUDE:

- Macro Nut Spread Range
- Macro Organic Peanut Butter
- Mayver's nut pastes and butters range
- Mayver's Original Super Spread
- Mayver's Tahini
- Sanitarium Natural Peanut Butter.

# Selection Criteria:
# Ready to Eat Meals

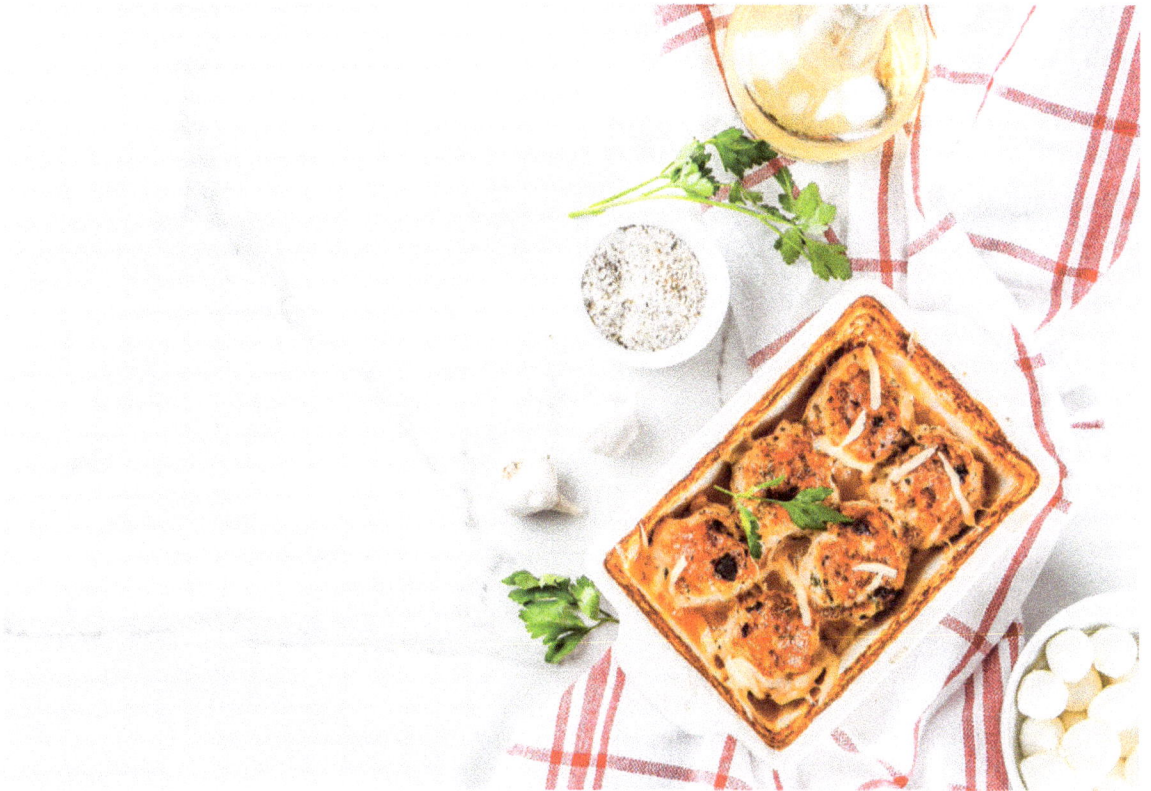

# Liquid Breakfast

In an ideal world, we should all be making time to sit and enjoy a nutrient dense breakfast such as cereal, fruit, yoghurt, eggs, grainy toast or beans. However for many people, this does not always happen, hence we have included this section on liquid breakfast options.

Many liquid breakfast options are low in protein and high in sugar, so be sure to use our selection criteria below.

Very low calorie products that come in powdered form to be mixed with milk or water are a good option to consider too, such as Formulite or Optifast.

These liquid breakfast options can make a great back up for those busy days, where breakfast otherwise would have been missed.

## NFWLS SELECTION CRITERIA

Due to the varied volumes of breakfast drinks, we suggest you compare per 100g (or 100ml). However, do keep in mind the portion you choose to drink. Some varieties come as a 400 – 500ml bottle, whereas some are smaller tetra packs. Larger volumes could be divided over two to three breakfasts, depending on the volume you tolerate. Always remember to stop at satisfied, not full.

## WHEN CHOOSING A LIQUID BREAKFAST, LOOK FOR OPTIONS THAT HAVE:

- Greater than 6g protein per 100g
- Less than 15g carbohydrate per 100g
- Less than 10g sugar per 100g
- Less than 5g total fat per 100g.

## OUR TOP PICKS INCLUDE:

- Formulite, made with water
- Optifast, made with water
- Rokeby Farms Whole Protein Breakfast Smoothie
- Up&Go Energize.

# Frozen Meals

When life gets busy and you need dinner in a hurry, frozen meals are one option to consider. However care needs to be taken, as many options are high in carbohydrate and salt and low in good quality protein and fibre.

Look for options that are based on protein and vegetables where you can.

You may find the full portion is too large, so try to eat the protein and vegetable components first, before filling up on the carbohydrate foods.

Before stocking up your freezer it is useful to become familiar with the following selection criteria to help guide your choice.

NFWLS SELECTION CRITERIA

WHEN CHOOSING A FROZEN MEAL, LOOK FOR OPTIONS THAT HAVE:

- Greater than 15g protein per meal
- Less than 30g carbohydrate per meal
- Greater than 6g fibre per meal
- Less than 5g total fat per 100g
- Less than 400mg sodium per 100g.

OUR TOP PICKS INCLUDE:

- Lite n Easy Chicken and Cashew Bowl*
- Lite n Easy Roast Chicken & Gravy (Lite Meal)
- Lite n Easy Pulled Texas BBQ Lamb (Lite Meal)*
- Super Nature, Super Protein Slow Cooked Lamb with Chickpea, Amaranth & Sweet Potato Mash**
- Woolworths Delicious Nutritious Beef & Tomato Casserole
- Woolworths Delicious Nutritious Asian Style Chicken.

Note: Lite n Easy is an online meal delivery service.

* Slightly below our selection criteria for fibre.
** Fibre content unknown.

# Fresh, Ready to Heat and Eat Meals

The range of fresh, ready to heat meals is expanding both in the supermarket and online.

These can make a good option for lunch or dinner and can certainly help reduce the need for traditional takeaway foods.

As with frozen meals, it is important you look for options that are rich in protein and fibre and not purely based on carbohydrate foods.

The following selection criteria can help guide your choice.

NFWLS SELECTION CRITERIA

WHEN CHOOSING A FRESH READY TO HEAT MEAL, LOOK FOR OPTIONS THAT HAVE:

- Greater than 15g protein per meal
- Less than 30g carbohydrate per meal
- Greater than 6g fibre per meal
- Less than 5g total fat per 100g
- Less than 400mg sodium per 100g.

OUR TOP PICKS INCLUDE

- Crudo High Protein Turkey Club Salad*
- Woolworths Delicious Nutrition Beef & Barley Casserole **
- YouFoodz Clean Chicken and Broccoli**
- YouFoodz Clean Chicken and Sweet Potato Mash**
- YouFoodz Clean Paprika Chicken
- YouFoodz Chicken Katsu Salad **
- YouFoodz Slow-Cooked Lamb Shanks **

Note: YouFoodz is an online meal delivery company.

* Fibre content unknown, slightly lower than our selection criteria for protein.
** Slightly lower than our selection criteria for fibre.

# Shelf Stable Meals

Shelf stable meals can make a handy pantry staple and an easy 'grab and go' lunch.

There are a lot of choices available, but many of these are too low in protein or high in sodium. It doesn't mean they have to be avoided, but must not be relied on to meet your nutritional needs.

The best options are rich in protein, not too salty and contain a good boost of fibre.

The following selection criteria can help guide your choice.

## NFWLS SELECTION CRITERIA

### WHEN CHOOSING A SHELF STABLE MEAL, LOOK FOR OPTIONS THAT HAVE:

- Greater than 15g protein per meal/serve
- Less than 30g carbohydrate per meal/serve
- Greater than 6g fibre per meal/serve
- Less than 10g total fat per 100g
- Less than 3g saturated fat per 100g
- Less than 400mg sodium per 100g.

### OUR TOP PICKS INCLUDE:

- John West Protein + Tuna and Bean Range
- Sirena Tuna and Bean Range.

# Soups

A quick, easy, warming soup in winter is a very popular lunch choice. Nothing quite beats homemade options, but in our time-pressured lives the convenience of store bought soups often wins.

Some commercial options are often little more than salty hot water, offering very little nutrition.

The following criteria can help guide you towards soups that provide a more nutritious choice.

NFWLS SELECTION CRITERIA

WHEN CHOOSING A SOUP, LOOK FOR OPTIONS THAT HAVE:

- Greater than 8g protein per serve of soup
- Less than 30g carbohydrate per serve of soup
- Less than 10g total fat per 100g
- Less than 400mg sodium per 100g.

OUR TOP PICKS INCLUDE:

- Campbell's Chunky Beef & Veg
- Darikay Hearty Chicken Soup
- Formulite Lupin Soups*
- Heinz Soup of the Day Pouch, Old Fashioned Chicken
- La Zuppa Hearty Chicken & Vegetable with Rice Soup Bowl.

* Formulite soups are available online. They are significantly higher in sodium than our selection criteria and are not suitable on a low sodium diet.

# Selection Criteria:
# Snacks

# Muesli Bars

Muesli bars can make a handy, portable snack when you are on the go.

However, some muesli bars are as high in sugar as your favourite chocolate bar! They can be the ultimate nutritional 'wolf in sheep's clothing'.

When selecting a muesli bar, try to ensure it has plenty of protein and does not contain excessive carbohydrate.

The following selection criteria can help you select a suitable option.

As protein bars are portion controlled, we suggest you look per serve.

### WHEN CHOOSING A MUESLI BAR, LOOK FOR OPTIONS THAT HAVE:

- Greater than 8g of protein per bar
- Less than 15g of carbohydrate per bar
- Less than 10g sugar per bar
- Less than 12g fat per bar
- Less than 3g saturated fat per bar
- Greater than 3g fibre per bar.

### OUR TOP PICKS INCLUDE:

- Carman's Protein Muesli Bar Range*
- Heritage Mill Roasted Nut Protein Bars
- Nice & Natural Protein Nut Bars
- Tasti Protein Muesli Bar Range* **.

* Slightly outside of our selection criteria in some flavours.
** Fibre content unknown.

# Savoury Snacks

We are often asked about portable savoury snack options. Unfortunately many seemingly healthy options provide little nutrition and have as much fat and salt as potato chips.

Don't be fooled by the packaging. Even if it claims to be vegetable chips, grain snacks or baked not fried, be sure to check the nutrition information panel to see if it is in fact a good choice.

When selecting a savoury snack, aim to select those lower in fat and salt and higher in protein and fibre.

### NFWLS SELECTION CRITERIA

### WHEN CHOOSING A SAVOURY SNACK, LOOK FOR OPTIONS THAT HAVE:

- Less than 15g fat per 100g
- Less than 3g saturated fat per 100g
- Less than 400mg sodium per 100g.

### AS A BONUS, ALSO LOOK FOR:

- Greater than 15g protein per 100g
- Greater than 6g fibre per 100g.

### OUR TOP PICKS INCLUDE:

- The Happy Snack Company Roasted Chic Peas, Lightly Salted
- The Happy Snack Company, Roasted Fava Beans, Pizza, Salt and Vinegar and Lightly Salted**
- Macro Air Popped Pop Corn, Lightly Salted
- Macro Cheeky Chickpeas, Lightly Seasoned*
- Macro Eda-Yummy Mix
- Macro Lentil Bites, Cruzin Carrot*
- Macro Sassy Chickpeas, Falafel Flavoured*.

*Slightly higher in fat than our selection criteria.
**Higher in fat than our selection criteria.

# Dips

When selected wisely, dips served with grainy crackers or vegetable sticks can make a healthy snack.

Unfortunately many commercial dips have up to 50% fat and can be high in salt, making them more of an indulgence.

The best dip is one you make yourself. Use a higher protein Greek yoghurt (see page 26) as a base and add grated cucumber, garlic and mint, or blend in beetroot and mint to make super simple, healthy options.

When selecting commercial dips, it is important to consider the fat and salt content. The following selection criteria can help guide your choice.

## NFWLS SELECTION CRITERIA

As dips are not portion controlled, we suggest you look per 100g.

## WHEN CHOOSING A DIP, LOOK FOR OPTIONS THAT HAVE:

- Less than 15g fat per 100g
- Less than 3g saturated fat per 100g
- Less than 400mg sodium per 100g.

## OUR TOP PICKS INCLUDE:

- Black Swan Skinny Hommus
- Black Swan Skinny Tzatziki
- Bulla Onion & Chive Cottage Cheese
- Doritos Salsa *
- Old El Paso Salsa *
- Yumi Baked Mediterranean Eggplant dip**.

* Slightly higher in sodium than our selection criteria

** Higher in sodium than our selection criteria, not suitable on a low salt diet.

# Selection Criteria: Protein Bars, Balls, Powders & Shakes

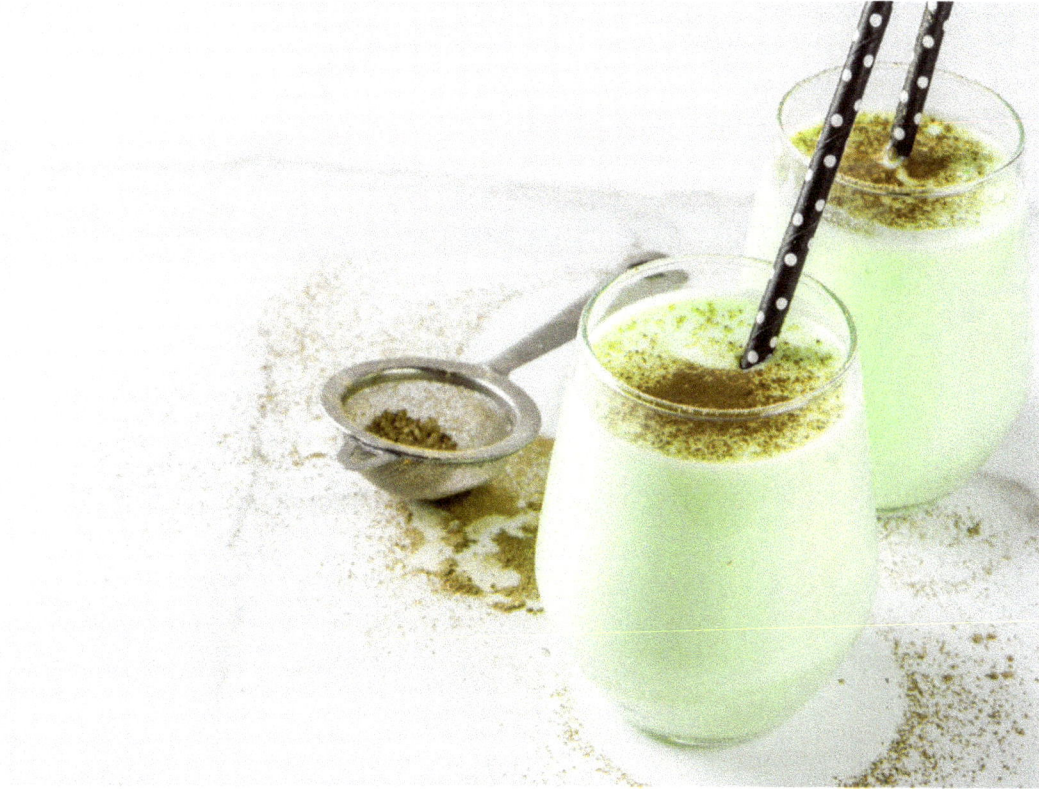

........................

# Protein Bars

Consuming enough protein post weight loss surgery is critical for your health and weight loss success, however this can be easier said than done. For this reason, many people look to commercial protein bars for a portable, portioned mid meal protein hit. Even so, they are certainly not an essential part of your post surgery diet.

Protein bars are highly processed, often with long ingredient lists, so not always suitable for those who prefer a whole food diet.

Protein bars often come with a high price tag, so if you do choose to include them, it is important you know what to look for to ensure you are getting the best value for money.

## NFWLS SELECTION CRITERIA

### WHEN CHOOSING A PROTEIN BAR, LOOK FOR OPTIONS THAT HAVE:

- Greater than 10g of protein per bar
- Less than 10g fat per bar
- Less than 10g carbohydrate per bar
- Less than 5g sugar per bar.

### OUR TOP PICKS INCLUDE:

- Body Trim Low Carb Protein Bar
- BSc High Protein, Low Carb Bar
- Optimum Nutrition Protein Stix
- Quest Protein Bar
- The Bar Counter High Protein Bar.

### A NOTE ON PROTEIN BALLS

Most commercially available protein balls are high in sugar, with up to three teaspoons of sugar per ball. If you are looking for a protein ball, aim for greater than 5-10g of protein, less than 20g of carbohydrate and less than 10g of sugar per ball.

Our top picks include Bounce Cacao Mint and Chia Almond flavours.

# Protein Powders

Protein powders are an effective way of boosting your protein intake without adding extra volume. This is particularly useful in the early postoperative period when your capacity is very restricted.

Unflavoured options are versatile and can be added into both sweet and savory foods and fluids.

Flavoured varieties can add interest into smoothies and shakes, and are a great base for home-made protein balls.

The best protein powder option following weight loss surgery is a whey protein isolate. Whey is the best source of Leucine, an amino acid that is important in muscle sparing, hence why it is our first choice.

If you don't like the taste of whey, egg white protein powders are also very high quality and are a good alternative.

If you prefer a plant based powder look for options based on a pea and rice blend as these contain the best amino acid profiles.

## NFWLS SELECTION CRITERIA

### WHEN CHOOSING A PROTEIN POWDER, LOOK FOR OPTIONS THAT HAVE:

- Greater than 80g of protein per 100g
- Less than 2g of fat per 100g
- Less than 2g of sugar per 100g
- A whey protein isolate base.

### OUR TOP UNFLAVOURED PICKS INCLUDE:

- Beneprotein
- Boomers WPI
- Bulk Nutrients WDP
- Cyborg Enhanced WPI
- Planet Food 100% Whey Protein Isolate
- Protein Supplies Australia WPI.

### OUR TOP FLAVOURED PICKS INCLUDE:

- Bare Blends
- Bulk Nutrients WPI
- Premium Powders Performance Nutrition WPI
- Protein Supplies Australia WPI.

# Protein Drinks

Ready to drink protein shakes can be found in the health food section of most supermarkets.

Like protein bars, they can be expensive, so it is important to look for options that best meet your post surgical needs

Protein drinks are not an essential part of your post surgery diet. They are a highly processed product, however can make meeting your protein needs easier in the early phases.

If you prefer to follow a more wholefood diet, you can make your own protein smoothies using milk, yoghurt, nut butters, seeds and fruit.

## NFWLS SELECTION CRITERIA

Due to the varied volumes in different protein drinks, we suggest you compare per 100g (or 100ml). However, do keep in mind the portion you choose to drink. Larger volumes could be divided over two to three serves, depending on the volume you tolerate.

## WHEN CHOOSING A PROTEIN DRINK, LOOK FOR OPTIONS THAT HAVE:

- Greater than 8g protein per 100g
- Less than 15g carbohydrate per 100g
- Less than 10g sugar per 100g
- Less than 5g total fat per 100g.

## OUR TOP PICKS INCLUDE:

- Musashi High Protein, Protein Shake
- Aussie Bodies Protein Revival
- Aussie Bodies Lo Carb Lean Protein Shake.

# Selection Criteria:
# Sauces, Condiments & Dressings

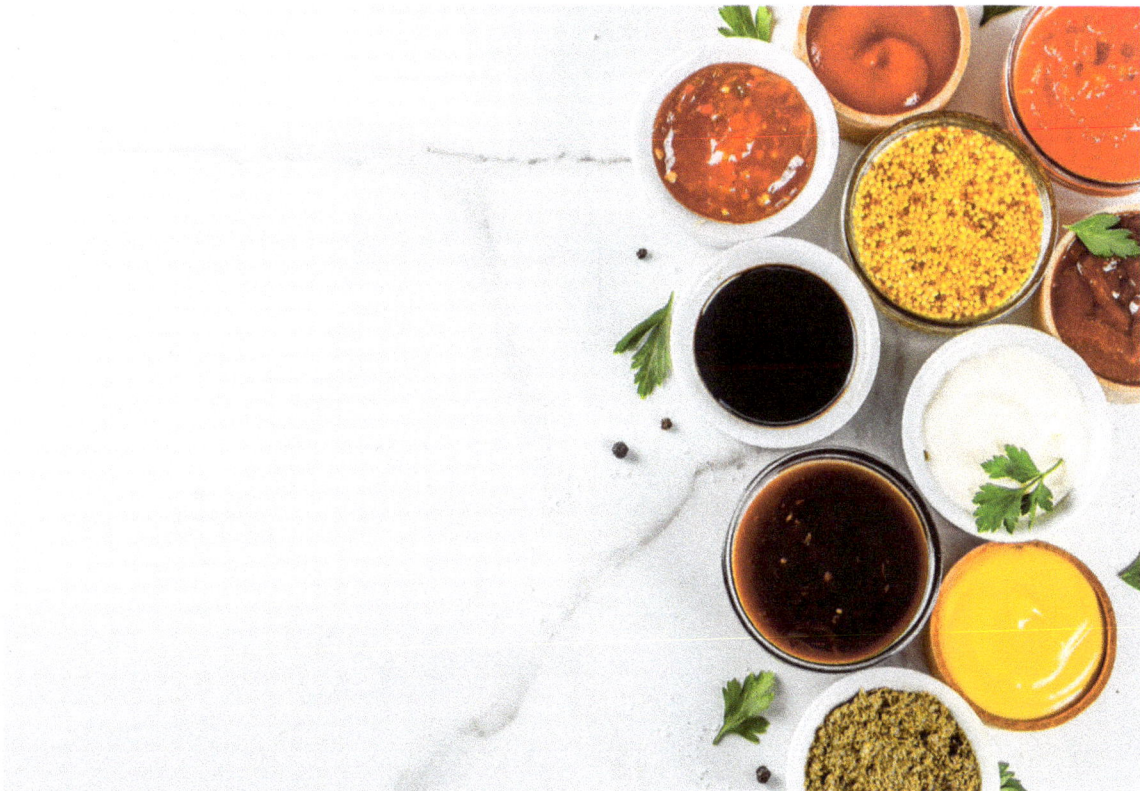

# Sauces, Condiments and Dressing

Sauces, condiments and dressings are a great way to add variety, flavor and moisture to your meals, which can also make eating more pleasurable.

For example, a salad dressing can help you eat more salad, and a sauce can make meat easier to tolerate, therefore they can help improve the overall balance of your diet.

Some sauces and dressings are high in fat, sugar and salt. However, given we typically only use a small amount of these, they are still suitable to include, just use the minimum amount you need to make your dish enjoyable.

Where possible, it is best to make your own sauces and dressings, so you can control exactly what is and isn't in them.

EXAMPLES OF SAUCES, CONDIMENTS AND DRESSING TO USE IN SMALL AMOUNTS INCLUDE:

- Vinegars
- Mayonnaise and salad dressings
- Pickles
- Chutney
- Relish
- Soy sauce
- Tomato sauce
- Worchester sauce.

# Cooking and Simmer Sauces

Cooking and simmer sauces make preparing casseroles, Bolognese, slow cooked casseroles and curry a breeze.

Care must be taken when selecting these types of sauces as the serve size consumed is larger than other side sauces and condiments. The excess fat, sugar and salt can add up.

Typically speaking, tomato based options are a better choice, but even these can be quite oily so it is still worth checking the nutrition information panel to ensure you are making a better choice.

### NFWLS SELECTION CRITERIA

As cooking or simmer sauces are not portion controlled, we suggest you look per 100g.

### WHEN CHOOSING A COOKING OR SIMMER SAUCE, LOOK FOR OPTIONS THAT HAVE:

- Less than 15g carbohydrate per 100g
- Less than 10g sugar per 100g
- Less than 5g total fat per 100g
- Less than 3g saturated fat per 100g
- Less than 400mg sodium per 100g.

### OUR TOP PICKS INCLUDE:

- Barilla Bolognese*
- Chicken Tonight Cacciatore
- Dolmio Extra Bolognese Pasta Sauce
- Dolmio Extra Tomato, Onion & Garlic Pasta Sauce
- Leggo's Pasta Sauce Bolognese with Chunky Tomato, Garlic and Herbs
- Masterfoods Curried Sausages Simmer Sauce*
- Sacla Italia Cherry Tomato and Roasted Garlic.

*Slightly higher than our selection criteria for sodium.

# Quick Label Reading Reference Guide

## Grains

| BREAD, WRAPS AND FLAT BREAD | |
|---|---|
| Carbohydrate | Less than 20g per slice/wrap |
| Protein | Greater than 3g per slice/wrap |
| Fat | Less than 5g per slice/wrap |
| Fibre | Greater than 3g per slice/wrap |
| Sodium | Less than 400mg per 100g |
| **CRACKERS AND CRISPBREAD** | |
| Protein | Greater than 6g per 100g |
| Fibre | Greater than 6g per 100g |
| Fat | Less than 10g per 100g |
| Sodium | Less than 400mg per 100g |
| **BREAKFAST CEREAL, PORRIDGE, OATS AND BREAKFAST CEREAL BISCUITS** | |
| Protein | Greater than 8g per 100g |
| Fibre | Greater than 8g per 100g |
| Sugar | Less than 15g per 100g |
| Fat | Less than 10g per 100g |
| Sodium | Less than 400mg per 100g |
| **MUESLI AND GRANOLA** | |
| Protein | Greater than 8g per 100g |
| Fibre | Greater than 8g per 100g |
| Sugar | Less than 15g per 100g |
| Fat | Less than 25g per 100g |
| Saturated fat | Less than 3g per 100g |
| Sodium | Less than 400mg per 100g |
| **RICE & RICE BLENDS** | |
| Protein | Greater than 4g per 100g |
| Fibre | Greater than 3g per 100g |
| **PASTA AND NOODLES** | |
| Protein | Greater than 6g per 100g |
| Fibre | Greater than 4g per 100g |
| Fat | Less than 5g per 100g |
| Sodium | Less than 400mg per 100g |

# Meat & Meat Alternatives

| DELI AND PRE COOKED MEATS AND SAUSAGES BURGER AND PATTIES | |
|---|---|
| Protein | Greater than 10g per 100g |
| Carbohydrate | Less than 10g per 100g |
| Fat | Less than 10g per 100g |
| Saturated fat | Less than 3g per 100g |
| Sodium | Less than 400mg per 100g |
| FROZEN CHICKEN, FROZEN FISH, SEAFOOD AND TINNED FISH | |
| Protein | Greater than 20g per 100g |
| Carbohydrate | Less than 10g per 100g |
| Fat | Less than 10g per 100g |
| Saturated fat | Less than 3g per 100g |
| Sodium | Less than 400mg per 100g |
| VEGETARIAN PROTEINS | |
| Protein | Greater than 15g per 100g |
| Carbohydrate | Less than 10g per 100g |
| Fat | Less than 10g per 100g |
| Saturated fat | Less than 3g per 100g |
| Sodium | Less than 400mg per 100g |

# Dairy & Alternatives

| COW'S MILK ALTERNATIVES | |
|---|---|
| Protein | Greater than 3g per 100g |
| Fat | Less than 3g per 100g |
| Sugar | Less than 5g per 100g |
| Added Calcium | Yes |
| YOGHURT | |
| Protein | Greater than 5g per 100g |
| Sugar | Less than 10g per 100g |
| Fat | Less than 2g per 100g |
| RICOTTA, COTTAGE AND CREAM CHEESE | |
| Protein | Greater than 10g per 100g |
| Carbohydrate | Less than 10g per 100g |
| Fat | Less than 10g per 100g |
| Saturated fat | Less than 3g per 100g |
| Sodium | Less than 400mg per 100g |
| ICE CREAM AND DAIRY DESSERTS | |
| Protein | Greater than 5g per 100g |
| Sugar | Less than 10g per 100g |
| Fat | Less than 8g per 100g |

# Ready to Eat Meals

| LIQUID BREAKFAST | |
|---|---|
| Protein | Greater than 6g per 100g |
| Carbohydrate | Less than 15g per 100g |
| Sugar | Less than 10g per 100g |
| Fat | Less than 5g per 100g |

| FROZEN MEALS, FRESH, READY TO HEAT & EATS MEALS | |
|---|---|
| Protein | Greater than 15g per meal |
| Carbohydrate | Less than 30g per meal |
| Fibre | Greater than 6g per meal |
| Fat | Less than 5g per 100g |
| Sodium | Less than 400mg per 100g |

| SHELF STABLE MEALS | |
|---|---|
| Protein | Greater than 15g per meal/serve |
| Carbohydrate | Less than 30g per meal/serve |
| Fibre | Greater than 6g per meal/serve |
| Fat | Less than 10g per 100g |
| Saturated Fat | Less than 3g per 100g |
| Sodium | Less than 400mg per 100g |

| SOUPS | |
|---|---|
| Protein | Greater than 8g per serve of soup |
| Carbohydrate | Less than 30g per serve of soup |
| Fat | Less than 10g per 100g |
| Sodium | Less than 400mg per 100g |

# Snacks

| MUESLI BARS | |
|---|---|
| Protein | Greater than 8g per bar |
| Carbohydrate | Less than 15g per bar |
| Sugar | Less than 10g per bar |
| Fat | Less than 12g per bar |
| Saturated Fat | Less than 3g per bar |
| Fibre | Greater than 3g per bar |

| SAVOURY SNACKS | |
|---|---|
| Fat | Less than 15g per 100g |
| Saturated Fat | Less than 3g per 100g |
| Sodium | Less than 400mg per 100g |
| Protein | Bonus – Greater than 15g per 100g |
| Fibre | Bonus – Greater than 6g per 100g |

| DIPS | |
|---|---|
| Fat | Less than 15g per 100g |
| Saturated Fat | Less than 3g per 100g |
| Sodium | Less than 400mg per 100g |

# Protein Bars, Powders & Drinks

| PROTEIN BARS | |
|---|---|
| Protein | Greater than 10g per bar |
| Fat | Less than 10g per bar |
| Carbohydrate | Less than 10g per bar |
| Sugar | Less than 5g per bar |
| **PROTEIN POWDERS** | |
| Protein | Greater than 80g per 100g |
| Fat | Less than 2g per 100g |
| Sugar | Less than 2g per 100g |
| Type | Bonus, a whey protein isolate base |
| **PROTEIN DRINKS** | |
| Protein | Greater than 8g per 100g |
| Carbohydrate | Less than 15g per 100g |
| Sugar | Less than 10g per 100g |
| Fat | Less than 5g per 100g |

# Sauces, Condiments & Dressings

| COOKING AND SIMMER SAUCES | |
|---|---|
| Carbohydrate | Less than 15g per 100g |
| Sugar | Less than 10g per 100g |
| Fat | Less than 5g per 100g |
| Saturated | Less than 3g per 100g |
| Sodium | Less than 400mg per 100g |

Photography: Shutterstock.

Graphic Design: Jayne Freeman.

www.nfwls.com